The Mindful Art of Himalayan Meditation

Susanna Qiang Huang

The Mindful Art of Himalayan Meditation

Susanna Qiang Huang

Copyright © Qiang Huang 2025

Published by 1st World Publishing
P.O. Box 2211, Fairfield, Iowa 52556
tel: 641-209-5000 ◆ fax: 866-440-5234
web: www.1stworldpublishing.com

First Edition

ISBN: 978-1-4218-3578-5

LCCN: Library of Congress Cataloging-in-Publication
Data

Table of Contents

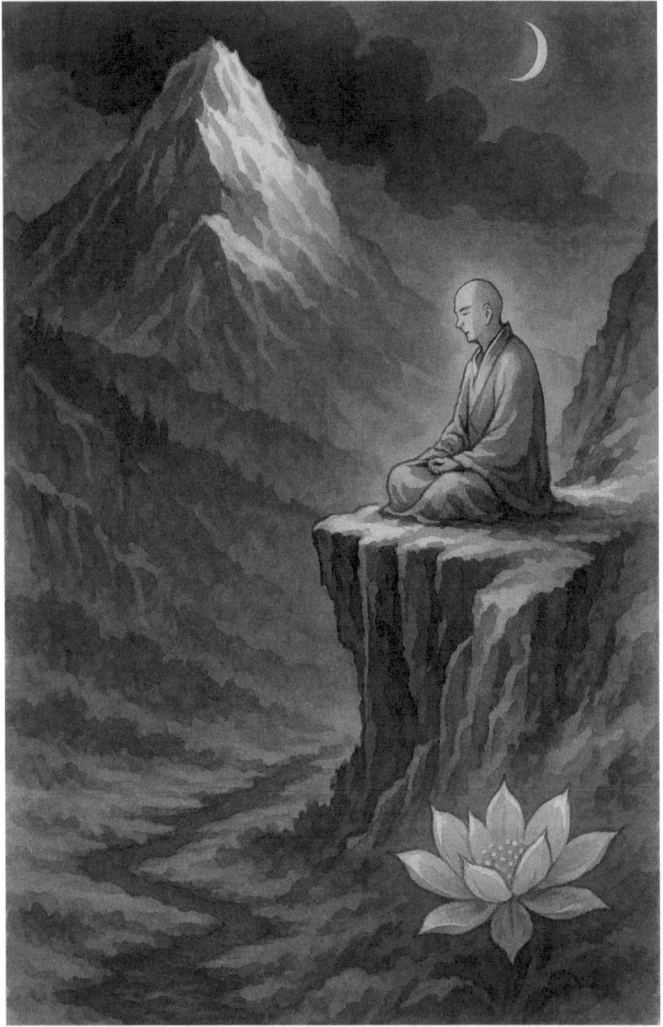

Preface

A Little Nepalese Boy in the Himalayan Mountains

"The affairs of the world will go on forever; do not delay the practice of meditation."
— Milarepa

In the beautiful Himalayan Mountains, a little boy was looking out through the window of his parents' house. The house was on the border of Nepal and China, in a blessed land often covered by white snow and dotted with wildflowers and animals.

This young boy was always meditating. There was no need to ask him why. His father was the local meditation teacher, as was his grandpa before him, his great-grandpa, his great-great-grandpa, and so on. This young boy spent quite a lot of time looking at the holy cave in the mountain from the window.

While other kids were playing freely, the little boy meditated and felt deep connections with the famous yogi, named Milarepa, who lived in this sacred cave more than one thousand years ago. Milarepa lived and meditated alone in the cave for years before he began teaching. According to folktales, he taught the art pf meditation to a deer, a dog, and a hunter. In the holy mountains blessed by Milarepa, there are still five streams where animals and people come to drink the blessed water. People have lived in this beautiful place for centuries.

Most people in the Himalayan region have special connections with Nature. Their lifestyles are always in harmony with nature, and very spiritual. In the past, there was no electricity. Now there are only solar-powered lights. Living in the snow-covered land since ancient times, Himalayan people perform special body movements and mind-taming exercises to generate inner heat and gain inner power and Qi. Unlike people doing yoga and meditation exercises in cities, Himalayan people practice yoga and meditation to survive. They are not just doing yoga to make their bodies look beautiful, especially in the winter snow, which is eight or nine feet high. You would agree that survival is more important, right? They also trained their minds in Love and Compassion.

This practice has a very beautiful lineage coming from the Buddha's teaching, and continues until now. Some Himalayan people keep their practices with special training secret. What we offer in this book are the Himalayan meditation practices for common people. It is a very beautiful concept.

What is Your Name?

"Knowing others is intelligence; knowing yourself
is true wisdom."
– Lao Tzu

Khenpo Karma Tenkyong, the little Nepalese boy, now a revered monk and teacher, started teaching us in his maroon robe at the tranquil Moon Creek Zen Garden. When Khenpo was a young boy, his parents sent him to be a monk, following the local tradition.

At the age of only 10, he went to India to study in one of the best monasteries in the country. Parents are alike, I thought, doing their best to plan for the bright future of their kids. Khenpo spent twenty-four years in India, much longer than his time in Nepal.

Studying under the guidance of the best Tibetan Buddhist teachers, he received a bachelor's degree, then a master's degree (I translated the degrees into terms used in universities). After teaching for another seven years, he was honored with the title Khenpo, a highly learned monk, akin to a professor at a university.

About ten years ago, he went to New York to teach. He talked to many people from all walks of life. It was a very different environment for a monk, who was used to a monastic life in India. He observed that many unhappy people had one similarity: they often looked outward, being constantly distracted by the outside, TV programs, games, and the latest fads.

He wanted to help people find happiness.

Back in the Moon Creek Zen Garden, he asked us to introduce ourselves by answering the following questions:

First Question: "What is the Name you'd like to be called?"

Second Question: "What is its pronoun?"

Third Question: "When did you go to bed last night?"

Fourth Question: "Tell us one good quality you have and one bad habit."

These are simple questions, easy to answer, right? Well, not really.

I found out that he designed these questions intentionally to bring people from looking outward to looking inward.

First Question: What is the Name you'd like to be called?

This immediately brings people's attention to themselves. "My name is Susanna Huang," I answered.

Second Question: What is its pronoun?

People see themselves through another person's eyes. "I'm she/her," I answered.

Third Question: When did you go to bed last night?

Why does he ask this interesting question? "I went to bed at 11 pm last night," I answered.

This question helps people notice their own activities, a very important practice.

Khenpo noticed that many American people slept late and woke up late. He asked us, "Do you notice there is day and night?" The nights are for people to recharge their Qi, vital life energy, much like we recharge our phones. At night, our bodies are healed; when we follow the natural rhythms, we are taking care of ourselves. When we go to work the next day full of Qi, we're less likely to be impacted by the negative energies around us. We bring good energy to our families and surroundings, making people happy.

It is our responsibility to take care of ourselves.

If we don't, who will do it for us?

If we take care of ourselves, we take care of others.

If we take care of others, we also take care of ourselves.

Fourth Question: Tell us one good quality you have and one bad habit.

When Khenpo talked to many students, he was surprised to learn that they didn't like themselves. When people focus too much on their bad qualities, they can easily get depressed. It is very important for them to see their own good qualities, from which they may have disconnected. We want to develop our good qualities and eliminate bad habits.

Through these four simple questions, our attentions were turning inward naturally.

Let's look at a fun bee picture together.

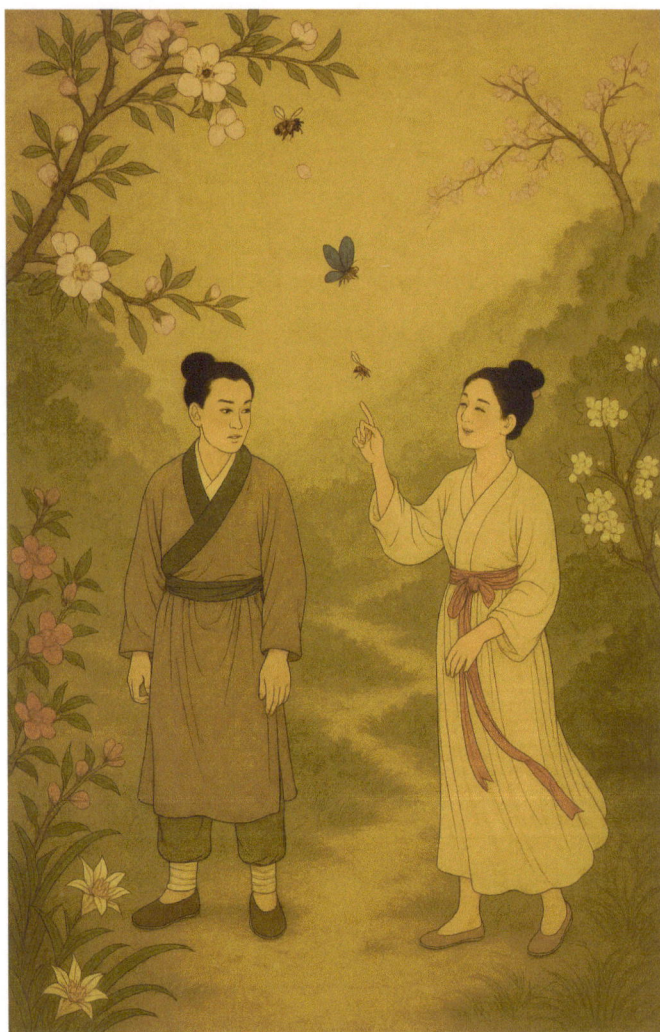

Are You Scared of Bees?

"Three things cannot be long hidden: the Sun,
the Moon, and the Truth."
– Buddha

Khenpo projected a picture on the white wall, a fun image.

In the upper middle, there is a bee, a live bee.

To the right stands a beautiful young lady looking up at the bee with a smiling face. It looks like she thinks the bee is lovely, with honey showing in her heart.

To the left stands a concerned man looking up at the bee with a scared face. It looks like he thinks the bee is going to sting him. He is scared.

Are they looking at the same bee?

They seem to be looking at two dramatically different bees—one bringing honey, the other bringing a sting.

They are living in their own worlds, unable to see each other.

But we know they are looking at the same bee; we are looking at the whole picture, unlike them.

Khenpo went on explaining, "We all have inner good qualities. When we are connected to these good qualities, we feel happy and see things positively. Very often, we have blockages, negative emotions, and obstacles inside us. When we are blocked from connecting to our inner good qualities, we feel concerned and see the stinging bee."

I looked at the picture, thinking, could the girl and the man look at the bee differently, even if they wanted to?

The young girl wants to be happy. The man does too.

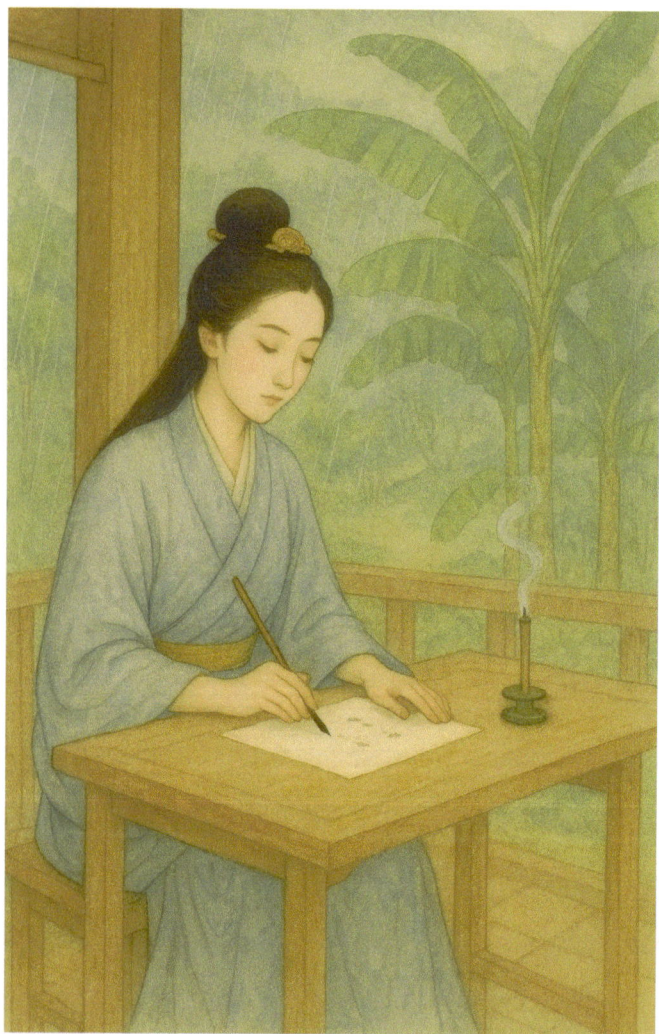

What is Meditation?

"The Moon, so pure. A wandering monk
carries it. Across the sand."
– Matsuo Bashō

Khenpo moved on, asking a new question, "What is meditation?"

I pushed away my reflections on the bee picture, ready to offer my thoughtful answers.

His question made me think of the day before, when Khenpo and I were at Bridge Park. It was a beautiful day: blue sky, white clouds, the river flowing among green trees, like an oil painting. There were many people on the bridge, enjoying the good weather.

I saw a smiling face walking toward me, the same smiling face of a short old lady I saw most days. She is my neighbor, taking a walk with her tall husband. I introduced Khenpo, who invited them to attend our meditation workshop. The tall husband politely declined, "I cannot even sit for an hour," he said. His leg seemed to have a problem, Khenpo observed.

At Moon Creek Zen Garden, Khenpo eased us into answering this question, assuring us that any answer would be okay.

"Silence," one person said.

"A group of people sitting together," said another.

Before giving his answer, Khenpo once again projected the picture of the bee, the beautiful young girl, and the concerned man. Now, a flashlight was shining on the picture, on the left, listing the positive thoughts, on the right, the negative ones.

If both could see the situation in the light, they would have different perspectives on the bee, the same bee.

Khenpo continued his teachings on meditation.

"Meditation is awareness. Meditation is knowing. Meditation is to become more familiar with the mind and how it operates. Meditation is the best method to be best friends with your own mind."

"What is the foundation of meditation?" Khenpo asked.

"That we want to do the meditation." My friend answered correctly.

"Yes. The foundation of meditation is that we have the intention to do meditation." Khenpo confirmed.

"So why is it that some people don't have the intention to do meditation? I thought to myself.

I suddenly realized that many people do not practice meditation because they have their own mental images of meditation, like the stinging bee image. They never challenge their assumptions about it.

I now understand that they were saying no to their ideas of meditation, not to the meditation Khenpo was teaching at Moon Creek Zen Garden.

Khenpo, although himself a monk, explained that we can meditate freely, not necessarily in a monk's way.

If somebody likes singing, when their mind and body are together, it is meditation.

If somebody likes drawing, when their mind and body are together, it is meditation.

I thought about my grandma. She was always sewing, peacefully. Her sewing was a beautiful meditation.

Golfing for somebody is meditation too if this person's mind and body are together, enjoying the sport.

When people make the wrong assumption about what meditation is, we often hear them saying, "I've never done meditation." Really? "I could not do meditation." Do you mean you could not sit long? Do you sing, draw, sew, or golf?

If they allow Khenpo to observe them for a short period of time, Khenpo may point out the moments they do meditation without knowing.

I remember a story in a book where a person asked a Guru, "When do you meditate?"

The Guru said, "Do you expect me to tell you that I meditate first thing in the morning, which you often hear?" The Guru continued, "I don't do that kind of meditation. I meditate anytime, in whatever I do, and wherever I go."

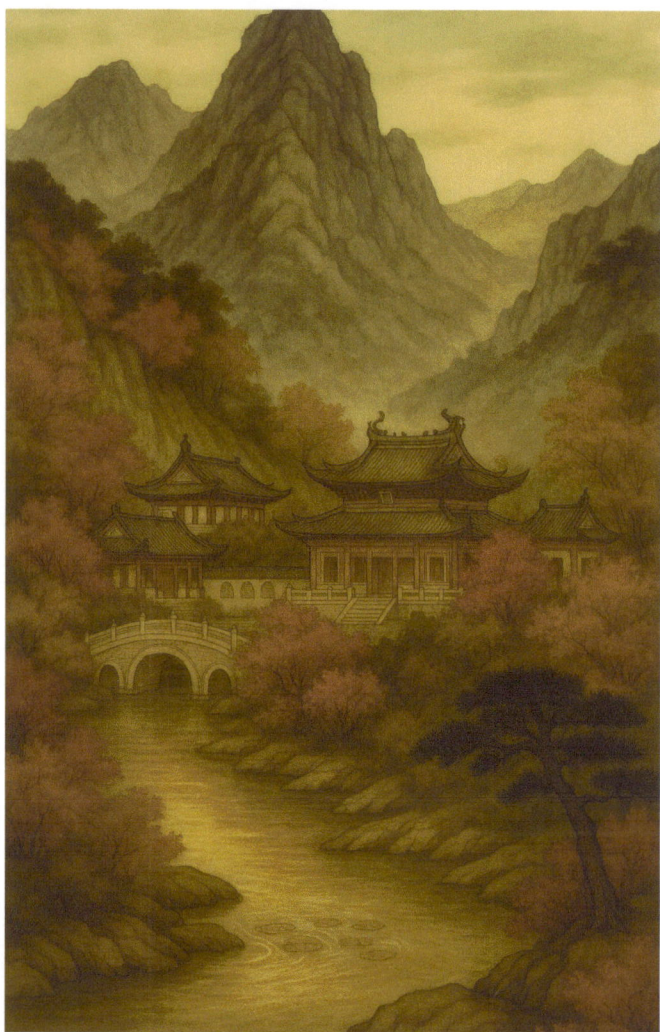

Why Do We Meditate?

"Happiness is the meaning and the purpose of life,
the whole aim and end of human existence"
– Aristotle

I picked up Khenpo from his hotel. On the way to the Moon Creek Zen Garden, we saw dead animals here and there. Feeling sad, Khenpo offered his prayers. I slowed down the car when passing by. This road sometimes had traffic, but not very often.

In the Meditation Room, Khenpo asked, "Would you want to have one part of the road clear of traffic, or would you want all the roads clear?" referring to our driving experience that morning.

"I want all the roads to be clear so I can get to where I'm going quickly," I answered.

This was just Khenpo's illustration, leading to a profound understanding of meditation.

He explained that, according to the teachings from his tradition, our body has 84,000 subtle intersection chakras. People often only know the Seven Main

Chakras or Three Main Channels.

If some of the intersections in our body are blocked, akin to experiencing traffic on the road, then oxygen will not reach these intersections. The brain would then have negative emotions such as anxiety and concerns.

So how is traffic related to meditation? I do meditation to be happy, while riding entrepreneur roller coasters.

Khenpo continued, "What are the five elements of our body?"

I thought it was Gold, Wood, Water, Fire, and Earth, from childhood learnings. It was a good try, but not correct.

Khenpo gave his Buddhist answer:

The first element is Earth. We're all living on Mother Earth.

The next element is Water. Our body consists mainly of water.

The third element is Fire.

The fourth element is Wind. Interesting. How is it related to the wind breathing meditation?

The fifth element is Space. More interesting. Is our body just like the sky, thoughts like clouds? I was curious.

We all have the same five elements. So, we are like everything else—the Moon, the Stars, the Universe.

When we take care of ourselves, we are taking care of others, and vice versa. It seems like deeper answers to why we meditate will reveal themselves slowly while we are learning a few meditation methods, such as wind, body, and mind.

Nine-Round Purification Breathing Meditation

"Purity or impurity depends on oneself. No one
can purify another."
– Buddha

Khenpo was teaching. He was firmly grounded. His
voice was deep and peaceful.

I could feel his beautiful energy enveloping our
tranquil Moon Creek Zen Garden.

"There are three parts to contemplate in meditation,
all three together, he told us:

"What Do We Do? – This is about our meditation
actions or movements."

"What Do We Think? – Our mind and body are
together, in Oneness."

"What Do We Visualize? – Let's look at the demon-
stration of Breathing Meditation Practice."

Khenpo demonstrated the Nine-Round Purification
Breathing Meditation first.

"Sit comfortably with your legs in the Lotus position and place your hands palms down on your knees. Your body is like a mountain, firmly grounded in Mother Earth."

I visualized myself as a mountain in the snowy Himalayan mountains in Nepal.

"Now visualize that you are sitting in front of a tree, representing your connection with the blessings from Mother Earth." I visualized a magnificent, beautiful tree in front of me, showering blessings of white light.

"When inhaling, you visualize the blessing white light from the tree filling your whole body, from the top of your head to your toes, cleansing your whole body. When exhaling, you visualize dark-colored coffee like smoke being washed away from your body. This represents your blockages, negative energy, and obstacles."

Our body has three main channels:

The Central Channel runs vertically along the spine and is Blue, like our Mother Earth.

The Right Channel is the channel of Solar Energy and is Red.

The Left Channel is the channel of Lunar Energy and is White.

Is our body like the sky, with the Sun, Moon, and Earth? I thought to myself, after listening to these names.

We do three rounds of breathing meditation practice on the Right Channel, then three on the Left Channel, and finally, three on the Central Channel.

Fold the middle and ring fingers and place the thumb on top of them.

Run the index finger slowly, tracing the Right Channel from the bottom up while inhaling deeply with loud nostril sounds. Then, turn the right hand, folding it down slowly to the knee while exhaling.

Run the index finger in the reverse direction, going up, making a small, beautiful circle near the nose, like receiving the blessings. Inhale and exhale deeply before touching the right nostril.

Press the index finger against the right nostril, blocking the air, and breathe deeply through the left nostril three times, making loud sounds.

Then, do the same with the Left Channel using the left hand.

Finally, do the Central Channel Breathing with both hands down on the knees.

Receiving the white light blessings from the magnificent, beautiful tree, I felt my body was purified, becoming cleaner and lighter with fewer blockages, negative emotions, and obstacles.

Walking outside the meditation room, I felt happy and peaceful under the blue sky, hearing the singing of the birds and the Moon Creek.

Vajra Wind Breathing Meditation

I like the Bell and Vajra, an advanced breathing meditation practice. Initially, I liked them just as Tibetan musical instruments, with their beautiful designs. Then I learned about their special meanings.

The Vajra, or Dorje, is a symbol of power and indestructibility. It represents the Method.

The Bell is a symbol of Wisdom. I like to listen to its sound, which dispels my ignorance.

The Vajra and Bell are often used together, symbolizing the union of Method and Wisdom in meditations.

Khenpo showed us the Vajra Wind Breathing Meditation Practice. It involves tracing the contour of a Vajra, experiencing its power with both mind and body together until we melt into this indestructible energy.

Sit like a mountain, firmly grounded in Mother Earth. You can imagine any mountain. I imagined sitting as one of the snowy Himalayan mountains in Nepal.

Relax both hands on top of each knee.

Visualize yourself sitting in front of a magnificent, beautiful tree, radiating blessings of white light.

The inhaling and exhaling breathing practice will purify your mind and body.

We will start with the right hand for ten times.

Fold your index and ring fingers, then place your thumb on them. Use your index finger to trace the left contour of the Vajra from bottom to top while inhaling, and continue to visualize. Inhale, breathing in the blessing white light into your whole body, from the top of your head to your toes.

Then bring your index finger down to trace the right contour of the Vajra from top to bottom while exhaling. Exhale, breathing out dark, coffee-colored smoke, representing blockages, negative energy, and obstacles.

Repeat this practice using the left hand ten times.

During this exercise, your mind and body are united, embodying the Vajra and its special nature.

Bell Wind Breathing Meditation

Khenpo then demonstrated the Bell Wind Breathing Meditation Practice.

It involves tracing the contour of a Bell, experiencing its wisdom with both mind and body together, until we melt into this energy.

Sit like a mountain, firmly grounded in Mother Earth. You can imagine any mountain. I was still visualizing myself as one of the snowy Himalayan mountains in Nepal.

Relax both hands on top of each knee.

Visualize yourself sitting in front of a magnificent, beautiful tree, radiating blessings of white light.

Inhaling and exhaling will purify your mind and body.

We will start with the right-hand for ten times.

Fold your index and ring fingers, then place your thumb on them.

Use your index finger to trace the left contour of the

Bell from bottom to top while inhaling, and continue to visualize. Inhale, breathing in the blessings of white light into your whole body, from the top of your head to your toes, filling your body, purifying all your subtle intersection chakras.

Then bring your index finger down to trace the right contour of the Bell from top to bottom while exhaling. Exhale, breathing out dark, coffee-colored smoke, representing blockages, negative energy, and obstacles leaving your body.

Repeat this practice using the left hand ten times.

During this exercise, your mind and body are united, embodying the Bell and its special nature.

Seven-Point Posture Body Meditation

When we train our body properly, it is easier to train our Monkey Mind. We need to find a good environment, have a comfortable seat, and maintain a good posture to practice. We could sit on a cushion, a stool, a chair, or a special meditation pillow. We were sitting comfortably on the cushions, while birds and the moon creek outside were singing together.

Khenpo emphasized the Seven-Point Posture of Meditation for good energy flow.

Sit with your legs in full-lotus posture, half lotus, crisscrossed on a cushion, or sit on a stool or a chair with balance. It is easy to find your stillness in your body when sitting on the secret chakra.

Place your hands in a meditative posture with your right fingers on top of your left fingers and your palms face up and thumbs touching. Place your hands about four fingers below your navel. Or you can touch your thumb to your ring finger, close your hands, and place

28

your hands on your knees.

Keep the spine straight so the central energy channel is loose and straight. This will help you make space for your monkey mind and keep the flow for your main channels.

Stick your elbows slightly out and make space for your shoulders.

Tuck the chin slightly into the neck.

The lips are also left to rest naturally, with the tongue resting against the palate.

Your eyes should be unwavering, focused on the space beyond the tip of the nose at a point 15 inches from your body. OR you can close your eyes. Practice compassionate eyes and a loving face.

We breathed in and out and noticed the sensation of the breath in our bodies. We were just noticing, just being aware. We breathed in long and breathed out long.

We could practice other forms of body meditation, such as mindfulness walking meditation, or standing meditation. Sleep is also meditation, the best form of meditation, my favorite.

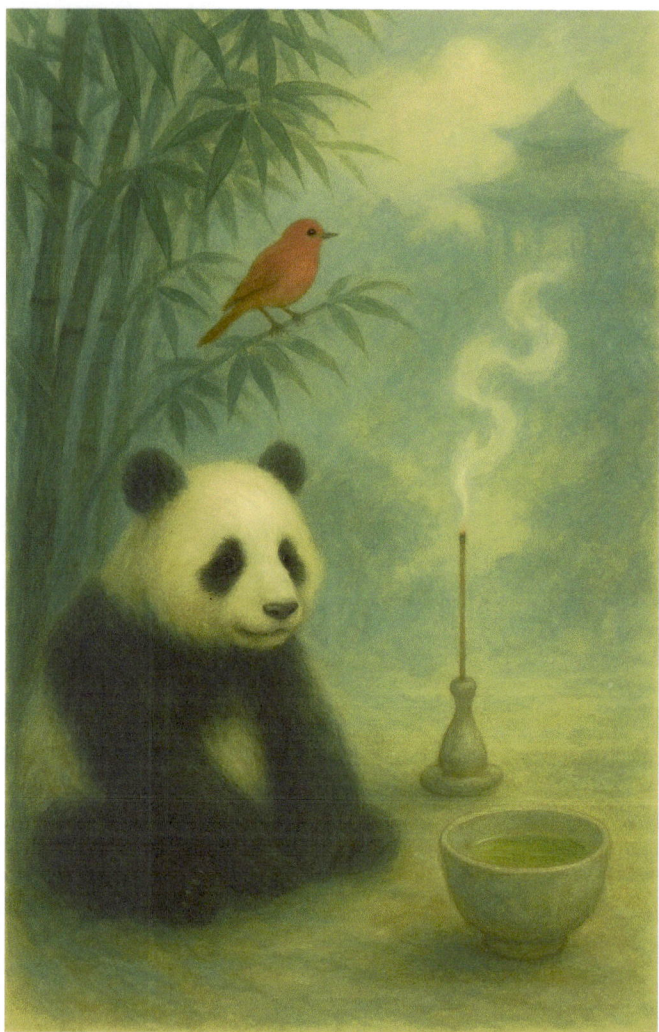

"Present" of Mind Meditation

"Yesterday is history, Tomorrow is a mystery."
– Former First Lady Eleanor Roosevelt

Most people who practice Yoga have beautiful bodies. However, Khenpo noticed that often their minds went somewhere else, going to their businesses or homes. Their bodies were in the Yoga studio, but their minds were not.

Khenpo explained that in traditional Himalayan Yoga and Meditation practices, the mind, breath, and body techniques are practiced together, inseparable. There is a Gift to live in the moment, not in the Past, not the Future.

We watched a cool short video clip from Kungfu Panda together.

Oogway, the great master, said to Kungfu Panda :

"Yesterday is history,
Tomorrow is a mystery,
but Today is a gift.
That is why it is called
the Present."

I took mental notes to use more of such video teaching tools in the future, as they are fun and easy to understand.

I received the present too. For instance, I love looking at flowers and taking pictures of them in all four seasons. In the mindful moment, there was no "I". I merged with the flower, and my surroundings disappeared. I was filled with joy and peace.

Khenpo shared a method to tell if our mind is living in the past, future, or present. Here it is:

If you're depressed, you're living in the past.

If you're anxious, you're living in the future.

If you're at peace, you are living in the present.

Train your mind to see good in any situation. You create your own story; be sure it is a good story.

Six Questions Asked Daily

"We are shaped by our thoughts. We become what we think. When the mind is pure. Joy follows like a shadow that never leaves."
— Buddha

Khenpo practiced and taught Love and Compassion in monasteries. But he was puzzled about why young people were not following their parents, coming to temples, not only in the United States, but also in his home country, Nepal, in fact, all over the world. Young people were avoiding religion, and at the same time, many of them were suffering.

In the old days, masters like Khenpo would sit on a tall seat, talking for hours, while kids were not allowed to ask questions. I haven't seen Khenpo sitting on a tall seat. He explained that he wanted to connect with young people to help them, and he went to New York Universities to study how to communicate with them.

Khenpo projected a quote on the white wall from The Age of Enlightenment, "The goal of meditation isn't to control your thoughts, it is to stop letting them control you."

There sat Khenpo, a Monk in maroon robes, with pure motivation of Love and Compassion in his heart, sharing his wisdom of meditation in English, using PowerPoint. He wanted to teach meditation differently.

Khenpo had asked himself the following six questions every day. He asked us this time.

First question: Why do you mediate?
"I've meditated over the last ten years to be happy in the chaotic business world," I answered.

"The purpose of our lives is to be Happy. Happiness is not something made. It comes from your own actions."

On the slides, Khenpo showed a few lines. He said, "meditation helps us experience true happiness, not temporary happiness, like that from a Coke bought by kids from the kiosks in their schools."

Second question: What is the meaning of meditation?
"Sitting is meditation" is a common assumption, but an incorrect one. Sitting is just the method, not meditation.

The meaning of meditation is to become more familiar with the mind and how it operates.

It is the best method to be a good friend with the mind, often called the Monkey Mind.

Meditation is awareness, like the flashlight, illuminating both our good qualities and bad habits.

It helps us work to bring more good qualities and

reduce bad habits and become enlightened.

Everyone's life goes up and down. That is the beauty of the art of life.

We often make up stories about things while living our lives. Our perceptions create reality.

Freedom is your power.

Knowing this is your power.

Meditation is knowing.

Third question: How do we meditate?

Monks and Nuns practice meditation in monasteries, but not many people can practice this way.

Meditation is, in fact, practiced across cultures by people from diverse backgrounds and religions.

Yoga meditation, popular worldwide, can also be traced back to its religious roots in the deep forest.

But over time, it seems some Yoga practitioners have started to only focus on body practices, alienating the mind.

Khenpo teaches Himalayan meditation, which originated from Tibetan Buddhism.

He said that all three—Body, Mind, and Breath—should be best practiced together.

Fourth question: Who should practice meditation?

The answer is everyone.

We all want to be happy, free from suffering.

Khenpo teaches meditation, not Buddhism, at many places, surprisingly in churches and schools.

Khenpo is particularly passionate about bringing

meditation into schools' curricula to help students.

It would be wonderful to teach more people Himalayan meditation, and I want to be part of this wonderful effort.

Fifth question: When is the right time to practice?

Practice meditation first thing in the morning and last thing before going to sleep. I sleep well after meditation. During the day, we can practice meditation when negative emotion arises or practice more often. The right answer is also anytime.

Sixth question: Where should we start practicing?

The answer is anywhere.

Sitting meditation is not the only method to meditate.

Meditation can be done when you're walking your dog, admiring the flowers, listening to music, writing a poem, playing an instrument, taking a photo, etc.

In other words: Anywhere!

Meditation is a way of living mindfully.

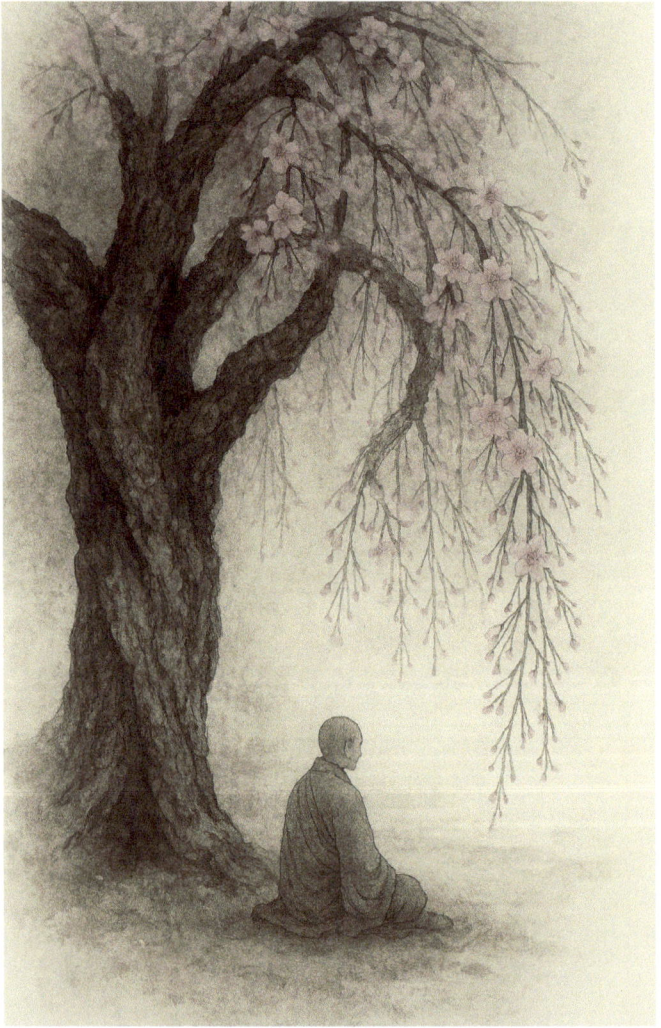

Practice Meditation in Your Daily Life

Khenpo shared the following to help us practice meditation in our daily lives.

First Step: Prepare your mindset to practice meditation.

Second Step: Find time for yourself to meditate. Can't find the time? You may want to read the "Why Do We Meditate" section again.

Third Step: If you know the Nine-Round Purification Breathing Meditation Practice, then practice this. If you don't know, breathe in long and gently for three seconds. Hold there for three seconds. Then breathe out long and gently for three seconds. Repeat five times.

Fourth Step: Practice the Seven-Point Posture Body Meditation. Be aware and notice each point to bring your monkey mind into your body.

Fifth Step: Focus with Mind Meditation. Be aware and notice your breathing in and out for twenty-one times. Alternatively, do Sound Meditation by listening to a mantra or music, or visualize and watch natural flowers. Practice calm tranquility meditation for 15–30 minutes.

Sixth Step: If you have a spiritual practice or individual practice, you can insert your practice here. Or you can do a mindfulness or healing mantra meditation practice ("Om Mani Padme Hum").

Seventh Step: Finally, dedicate your practice to yourself, your family, your country, to this beautiful Mother Earth, and to all sentient beings.

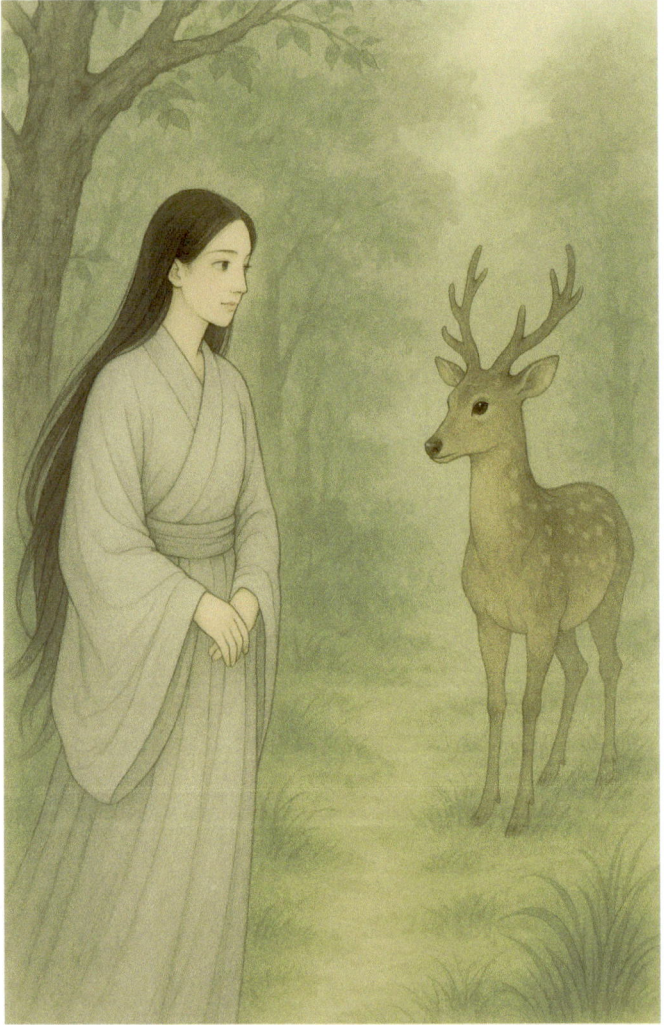

Deer and Bee,
The Final Chapter

"You are not a drop in the ocean. You are the
entire ocean in a drop."
— Rumi

Generosity is a virtue in many traditions.

I heard Khenpo say, not just once,

"You shall take care of yourself."

"It is your responsibility to take care of yourself."

"If you don't take care of yourself, who will?"

I was a little lost, especially since these words came
from a Monk. I meditated on these two seemingly con-
flicting views, taking care of others vs. taking care of
oneself.

Flowers always give me inspiration. I thought about
flowers. I love flowers, looking at them and smelling
their fragrance. In the snowy days, the flowers in my
garden died. If the flowers in the gardens of our hearts
wither, nothing can offer fragrance to people passing by.

If we don't take care of ourselves, akin to letting the flowers in the gardens of our hearts wither, how can we be generous, with no fragrance to offer?

Khenpo continued his teaching, "Meditation is the best method to make friends with ourselves."

We are sometimes like onions, wearing layers of masks. Not only could others not get a peek inside us, but we ourselves might also put masks on our true selves. If we don't even know ourselves, how can we distance ourselves from the harmful environment?

How can we intentionally put ourselves into a nurturing environment?

If we don't understand ourselves, how can we truly understand others?

How do we know that what we offer to others in "generosity" is perceived as helpful?

Through meditation, we can be best friends with ourselves, not using others to fill our emotional holes.

It is such a beautiful experience to be alone but not lonely.

Khenpo's teaching makes more sense to me now.

When you take care of yourself, you take care of others.

When you take care of others, you also take care of yourself.

Now I remember that we all have the same five elements: Earth, Water, Fire, Wind, and Space.

Khenpo teaches about Oneness in his language.

Khenpo wants us to meditate clearly with pure intentions.

I meditated diligently after he left Moon Creek Zen Garden. Interestingly, I not only felt more energetic and happier every day, I even lost some weight without changing my routines, and I felt younger. I also began to make business decisions with a clear mind and confidence.

This morning, I went for a walk with my puppy Otis, who suddenly barked.

I saw a deer looking at me from under the tree on the green lawn. We were so close, I looked directly into its beautiful almond-shaped eyes, feeling the tenderness of compassion flowing from it into my heart.

A few minutes later, a mom with a young kid from our neighborhood came by. She kindly warned me,

"I saw a deer following me. I am so afraid it will attack us."

I reassured her, "No worries. It is the same deer I saw just now. It really likes you, so it is following you."

I should have also told her that Deer are auspicious animals, embodying inspirational qualities such as love and compassion and harmony with nature. But I didn't go that far. She smiled and relaxed, continuing her morning walk with her baby.

I know the Deer is not the Bee in the picture that Khenpo showed us earlier. Still, I passed the honey from my heart, gained through meditation, to my neighbor to make her happier.

About the Author

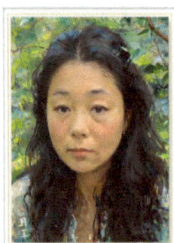

Susanna Qiang Huang (Yuexi) is a poet, writer, management consultant and contemplative practitioner whose journey bridges the worlds of strategy, spirit, and poetic insight. A student of Himalayan meditation, Buddhist wisdom, Daoist teachings, and Zen practices, she has cultivated a deep personal practice shaped by years of meditative study and inner stillness. Born in China and now living in a wooded Zen sanctuary near a golf course in Ohio, she writes and teaches from a space of serenity and awakening. Her previous works include *Moon Creek*, a collection of Zen poetry, and *Little Stone Lion*, a business book blending Eastern wisdom with Western strategies and purposeful leadership. In *The Mindful Art of Himalayan Meditation*, Yuexi offers gentle reflections and heartfelt guidance for readers from all walks of life who long for moments of inner calm, clarity, and happiness—anywhere, anytime.